Eloisa Andrade De Paula
Rayssa Ribeiro Marchioro
Daniele Antonio Schwarz

# Indirect Restorations in Dentistry

**Eloisa Andrade De Paula**
**Rayssa Ribeiro Marchioro**
**Daniele Antonio Schwarz**

# Indirect Restorations in Dentistry

## Ultra-thin Ceramic Veneers and CAD/CAM System

**ScienciaScripts**

**Imprint**

Any brand names and product names mentioned in this book are subject to trademark, brand or patent protection and are trademarks or registered trademarks of their respective holders. The use of brand names, product names, common names, trade names, product descriptions etc. even without a particular marking in this work is in no way to be construed to mean that such names may be regarded as unrestricted in respect of trademark and brand protection legislation and could thus be used by anyone.

Cover image: www.ingimage.com

This book is a translation from the original published under ISBN 978-620-2-04740-1.

Publisher:
Sciencia Scripts
is a trademark of
Dodo Books Indian Ocean Ltd. and OmniScriptum S.R.L publishing group

120 High Road, East Finchley, London, N2 9ED, United Kingdom
Str. Armeneasca 28/1, office 1, Chisinau MD-2012, Republic of Moldova, Europe
Printed at: see last page
ISBN: 978-620-8-16574-1

# SUMMARY

## 1. INTRODUCTION

The quest to automate all sectors of production is increasing, and dentistry is no different. As such, the manual procedures carried out in the laboratory stages for making prosthetic parts are increasingly losing ground to the advance of technology, which justifies this statement with the creation of the CAD-CAM (Computer Aided Design/ Computer Aided Manufacturing) system, one of the aims of which is to optimise the dental surgeon's clinical time. The term CAD refers to the design of a prosthetic structure on a computer using software, where the information is transmitted to the CAM system 1,2,3 for the manufacture of the same part by a milling machine.

This system was introduced to dentistry in 1971 by François Duret in France,4 and in 1980 it was perfected by Werner Mormann and Marco Brandestini in Switzerland and marketed under the name CEREC (Sirona® Dental Systems, Zurich, Switzerland), 2,5 short for Chairside Economical Restorations Esthetic Ceramic.

CEREC has automated the manufacture of prosthetic parts using prefabricated ceramic blocks made of zirconia, alumina and lithium disilicate6, which are milled to the millimetre in between 10 and 15 minutes depending on the size and type of prosthetic part to be made. This considerably reduces time when compared to manual fabrication by the prosthodontist, which can take 5,6,7 minutes.
hours or days.

In addition to the CEREC system (Sirona Dental Systems, Zurich, Switzerland), the Lava (3M ESPE, Germany), Procera (Nobelbiocare AB, Sweden) and Artica (KaVo Dental GmbH, Germany) systems, among others, are also available on the market today. All of these machines work using the CAD-CAM system and what differentiates them are their indications according to the type of fixed prosthesis to be milled, varying the number of elements and flexural strength.

number of elements and the flexural strength of the ceramics used, which range from 360 MPa to 1200 MPa. 8[1,3,]

Therefore, the aim of this study is to provide, through a case report, information on the CEREC CAD-CAM system (Sirona® Dental Systems, Zurich, Switzerland), its advantages and disadvantages and mode of operation for milling lithium disilicate ceramic blocks.

## 2. CASE REPORT

R.R.M., a 49-year-old female patient, after orthodontic treatment had been completed, sought aesthetic restorative dental treatment because she was unhappy with the size of her upper anterior teeth. She considered them to be small as a result of wear caused by bruxism (Figure 1).

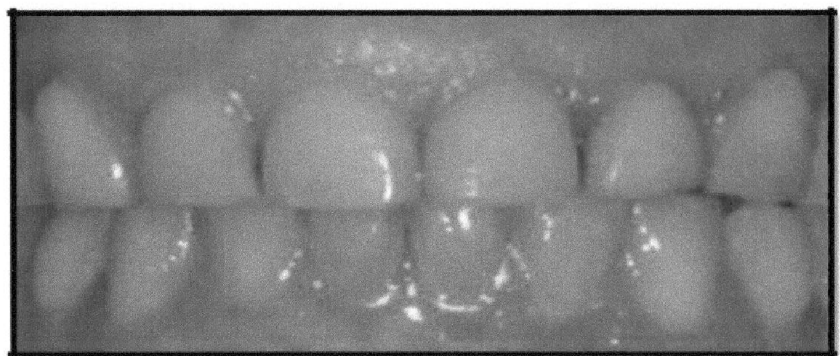

Figure 1

## 2.1. DIAGNOSIS

In the initial clinical examination, together with periapical radiographic and photographic examinations, it was observed that the elements in question were intact and had

feldspathic ceramic veneers made 13 years ago using the CEREC 1 system and without endodontic treatment. There was no incisal guide, no canine guide and the midlines were not coincident. Facial analysis from the frontal view showed passive lip sealing, without exposure of the upper incisors and the lateral view showed a good relationship between the maxilla and mandible, denoting a harmonious profile.

## 1.1. TREATMENT PLAN

It was proposed to make lithium disilicate ceramic veneers for teeth 13 to

23, made on the CAD-CAM CEREC 4 system - Software SW 4.2 (Sirona

Dental Systems, Zurich, Switzerland).

## 1.2. STUDY MODELS AND DIAGNOSTIC WAXING

Firstly, the upper and lower arches were moulded to obtain a study model. This model allows three-dimensional visualisation of the patient's teeth and occlusion. This same model was sent to the prosthodontist to make the diagnostic wax-up.

## 1.3. INTRAORAL DIAGNOSTIC RESTORATIVE TEST OR MOCK-UP.

The prosthodontist makes two copies of the diagnostic wax-up with the heavy addition silicone paste. One of the copies will be used to make the mock-up by inserting the bis-acrylic resin Protemp™ 4 (3M ESPE) into the transfer guide and taking it directly to the patient's mouth. In a few minutes, the silicone is removed and the simulation of the proposed treatment remains in the mouth.

In the second copy, a matrix will be made to guide the thickness and specific locations to be worn during tooth preparation, allowing the preservation of healthy tooth structure.

## 1.4. MAKING THE DENTAL PREPARATION AND WORKING MODEL

After seeing the aesthetic result and the patient's approval, the teeth included in the treatment were prepared for indirect veneers (Figure 2) and the upper and lower arches were moulded with silicone (two-stroke technique) to make the working model, using a double wire.

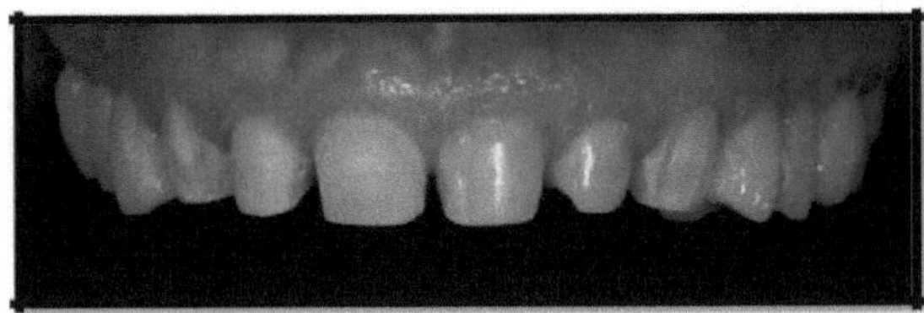

Figure 2

## 1.5. STAGES OF MANUFACTURING RESTORATIONS USING THE CAD-CAM PROCESS

The CAD project was started (Figure 3), defining the work as a biogeneric copy of the diagnostic wax-up and the type of restoration as *veneers,* selecting elements 13 to 23 (Figure 4).

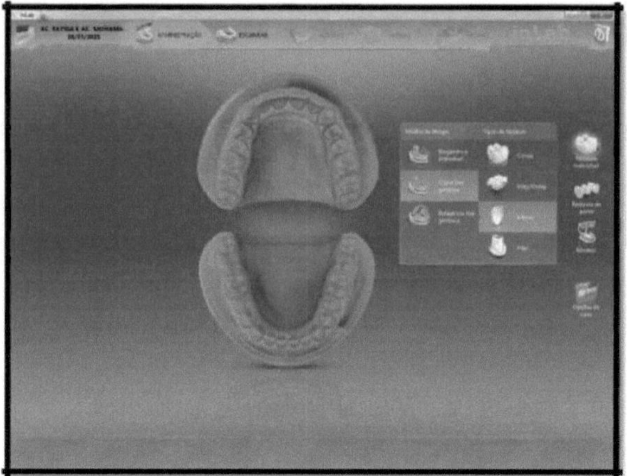

Figure 3

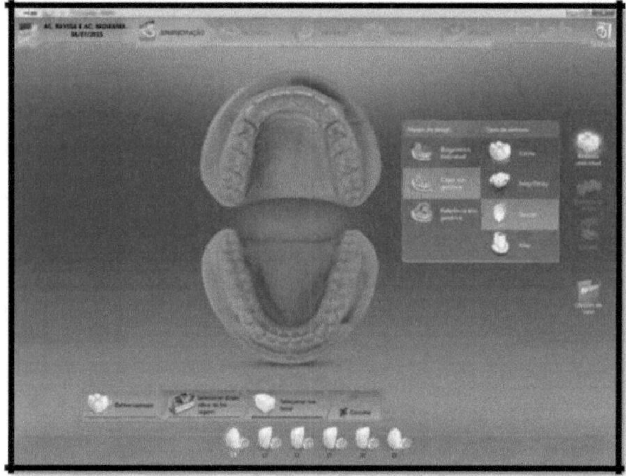

Figure 4

## 2.6.1. INDIRECT DIGITISATION OF THE PROSTHETIC PREPARATION

The CEREC Omnicam scanner (Sirona® Dental Systems, Zurich, Switzerland) was used to scan and copy the diagnostic wax-up (Figure 5), the tooth preparations on the upper working model, the antagonist arch of the lower model and the patient's occlusion (Figure 6).

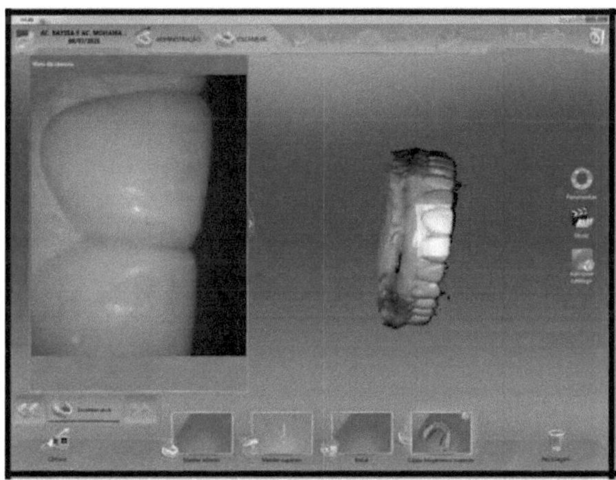

Figure 5

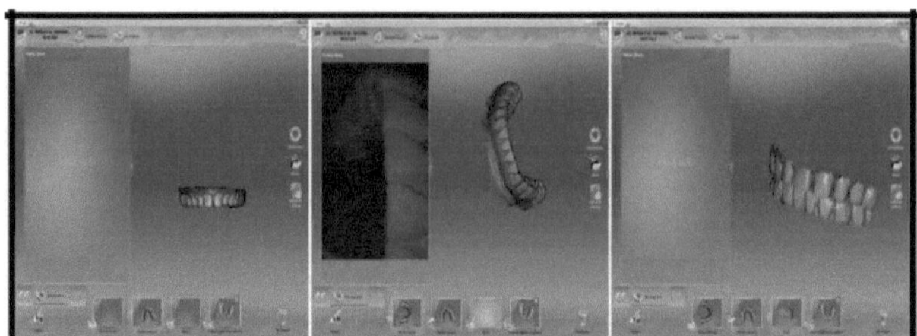

Figure 6

Based on this data, the software generates the upper and lower 3D virtual models (Figure 7) to check the model's axis, virtual definition of the midline and occlusal line (Figure 8) and the patient's occlusion (Figure 9).

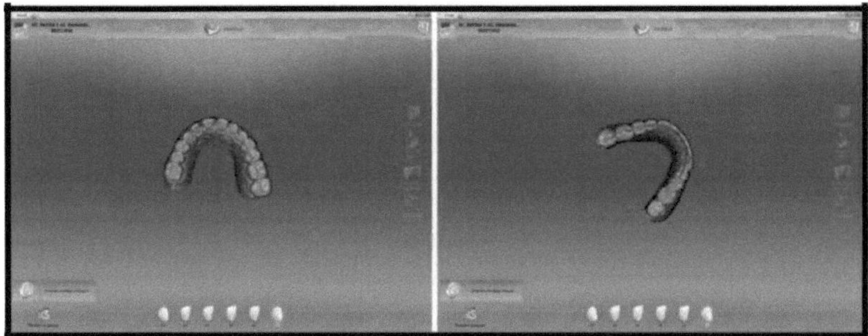

Figure 7

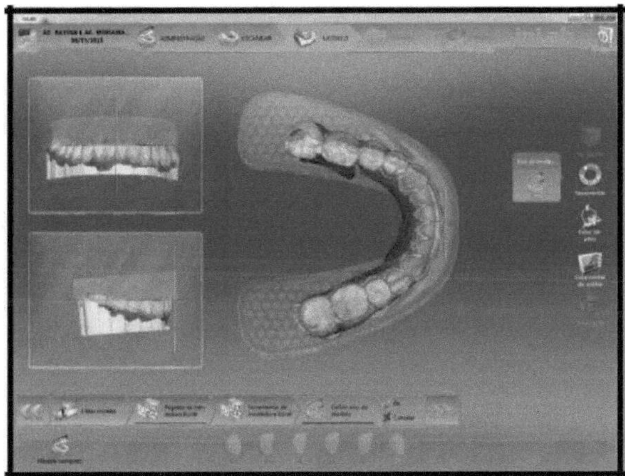

Figure 8

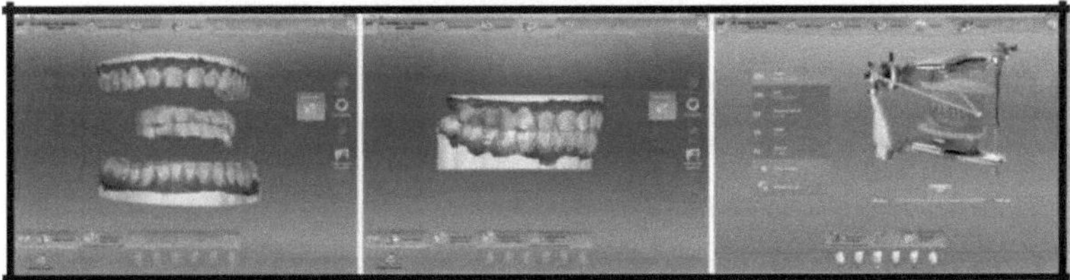

Figure 9

## 1.5.2. VIRTUAL DESIGN (CAD PHASE)

With the models obtained, the dies of each prepared element were virtually cut out to make the individual parts (Figure 10). The prosthetic margins were outlined (Figure 11), followed by the definition of the restoration's insertion axis on the virtual model, so that the diamond tip of the milling machine could mill all the angles of the ceramic block (Figure 12).

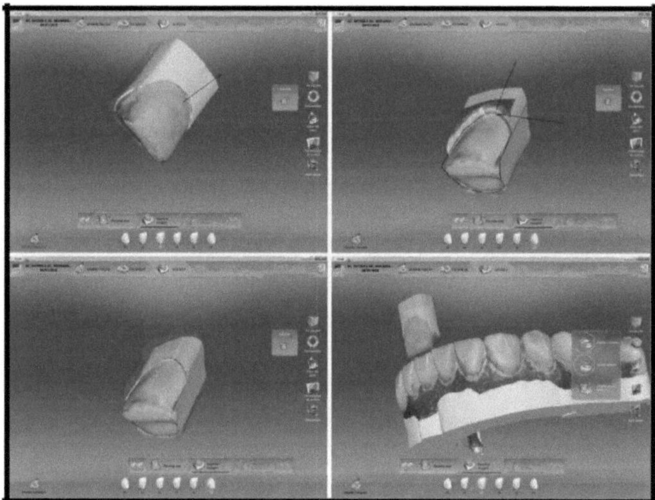

Figure 10

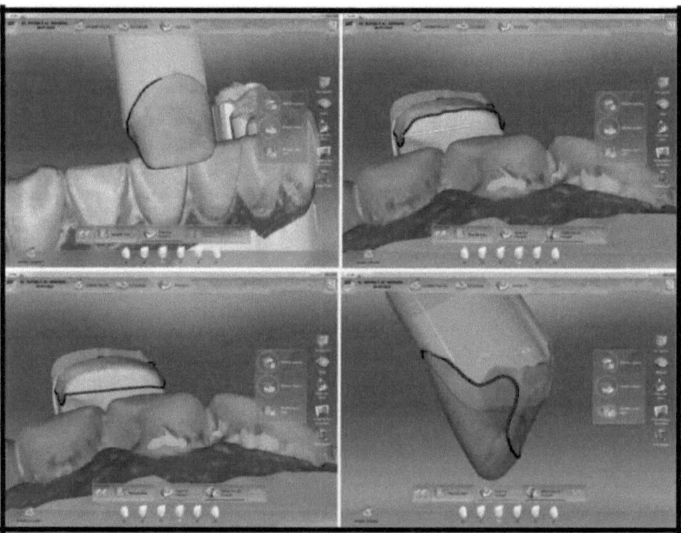

Figure 10

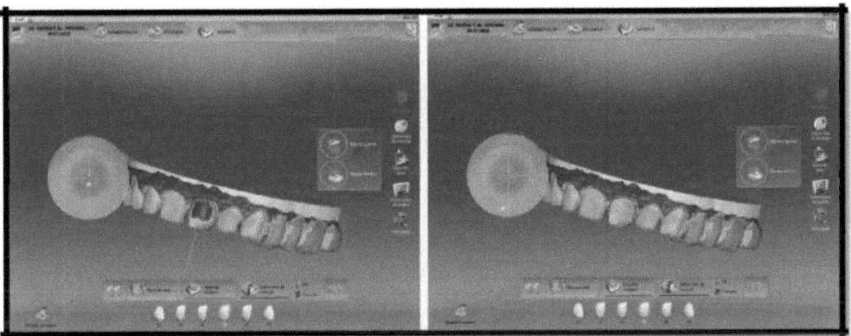

Figure 12

The restoration parameters are divided into 6 functions to generate a *veneer* proposal for each of the selected elements: 1. Spacer (set to 80 pm), 2. *Veneer* thickness (set to 300 pm), 3. Occlusal milling offset (set to 0 pm), 4. Margin thickness (set to 0 pm), 5. Instrument geometry and 6. Remove undercuts (the last two being set to "Yes") (Figure 13). With all the parameters set, the software generated a facet proposal for each of the selected elements (Figure 14).

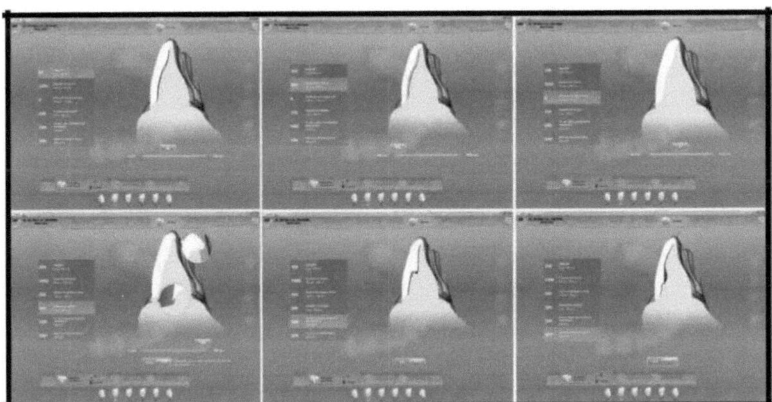

Figure 13

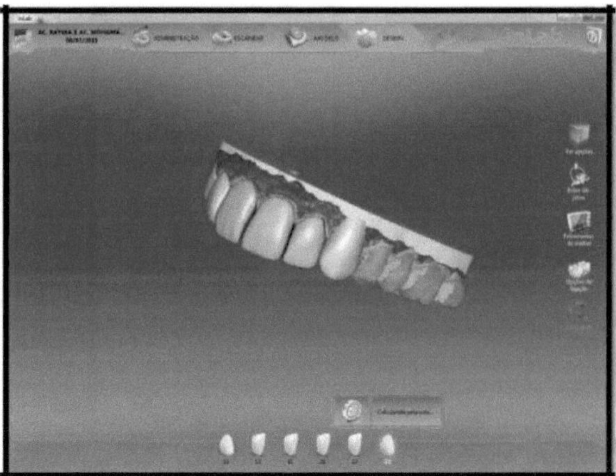

Figure 14

The software provides options for editing the pieces, such as shape, width, height, contact points and inserting or removing material (Figure 15), but as it is a copy of the diagnostic wax-up, it was not necessary to make any changes to the virtual *veneers*.

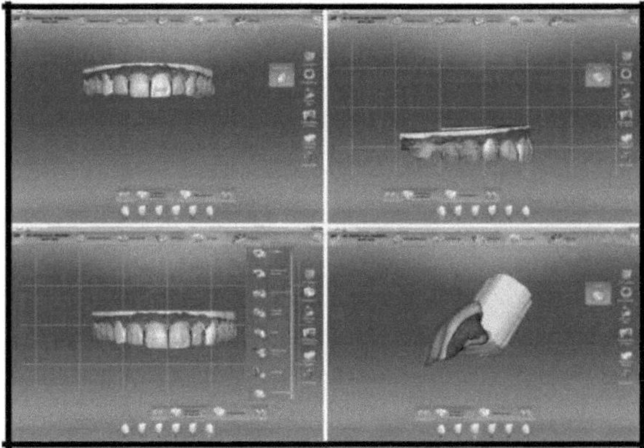

Figure 15

### 1.5.3.  CATERING PRODUCTION (CAM PHASE)

Once the part was ready in CAD (Figure 16), the six IPS e-max CAD HT (high translucency)

lithium disilicate ceramic blocks, A2 shade and C14 size (Ivoclar-Vivadent) were selected

(Figure 17), which were attached to the milling machine, one at a time (Figure 18), the position

of the veneer on the block was virtually defined and then the design sent to the CEREC MCXL

milling machine (Sirona Dental Systems) (Figure 19).

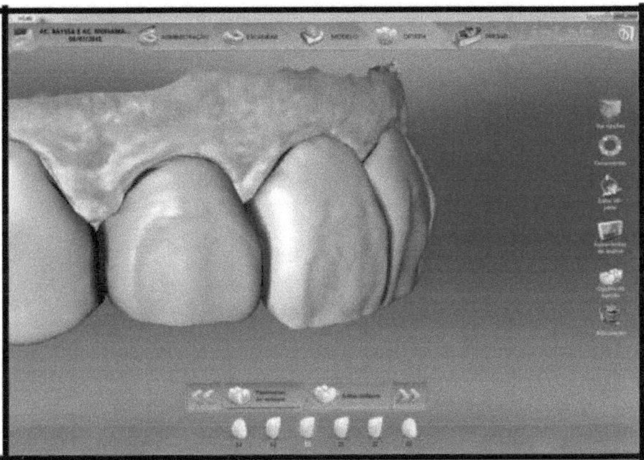

Figure 16

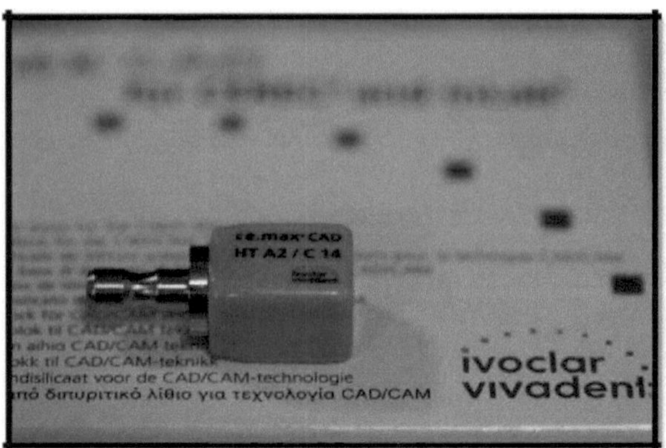

Figure 17

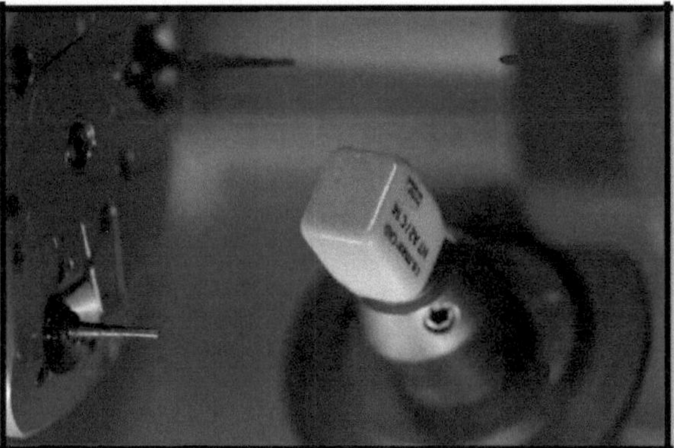

Figure 18

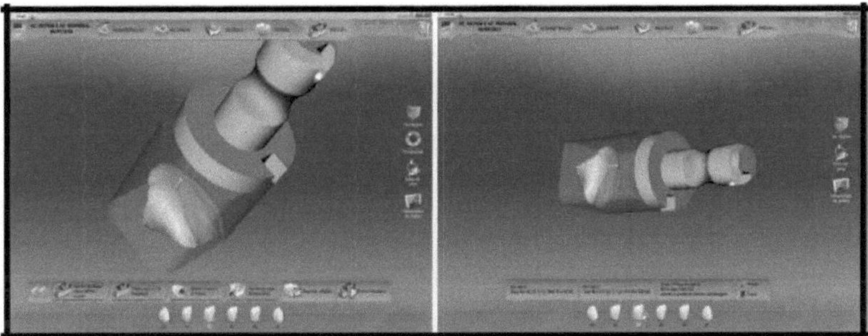

Figure 19

After an average of 12 minutes of milling each block, the six veneers were obtained (Figure 20), which were separated from the blocks (Figure 21) and given anatomical characterisation with a diamond disc and internal polishing with a rubber disc (Figure 22). Each piece was taken to the ceramic furnace to crystallise completely at a temperature of 840°C for a period of 25-30 minutes (Figure 23). After crystallisation, the pieces were made up with ceramic, glazed and sent back to the ceramic kiln (Figure 24).

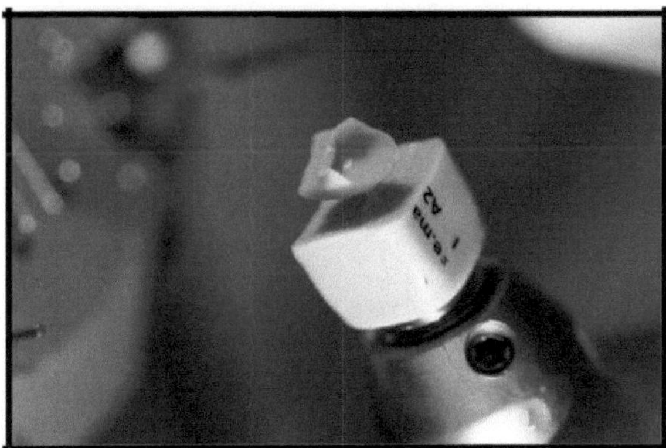

Figure 20

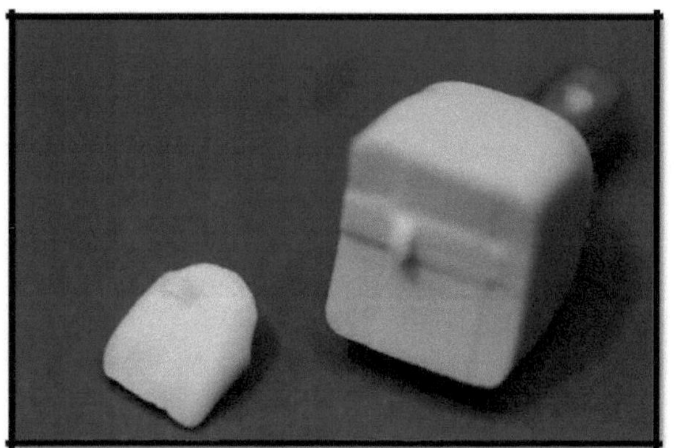

Figure 21

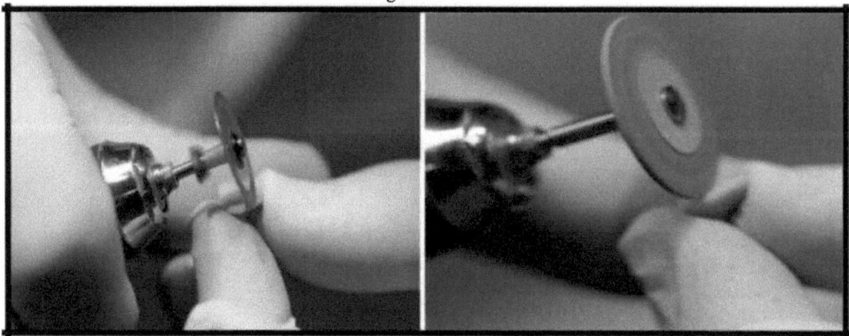

Figure 22

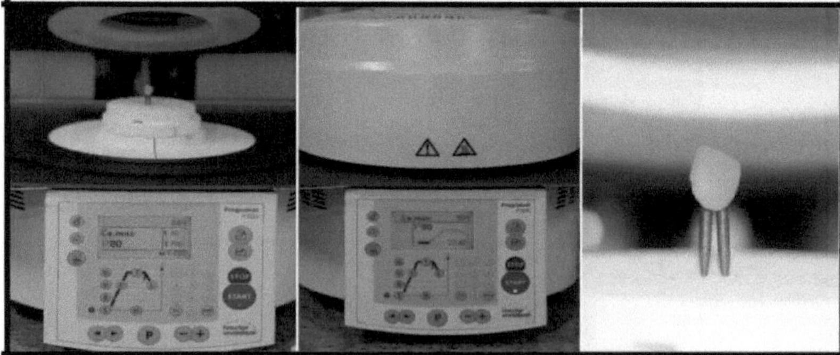

Figure 23

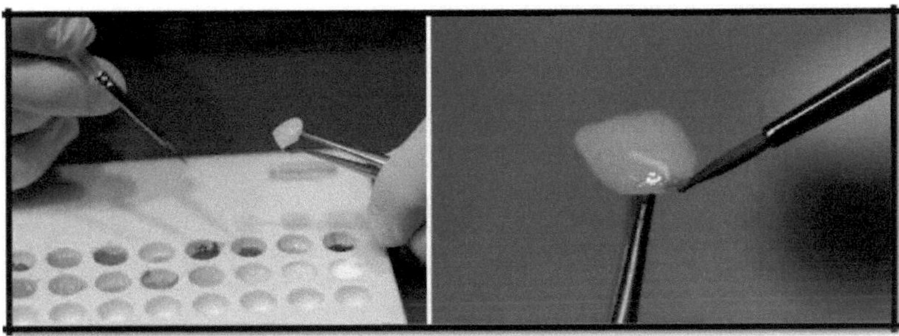

Figure 24

Once the pieces were ready (Figure 25), they were tested in the mouth using the Variolink Veneer cement try-in paste (Ivoclar-Vivadent, Germany) and the 110/A1 (White) shade material was chosen (Figure 26).

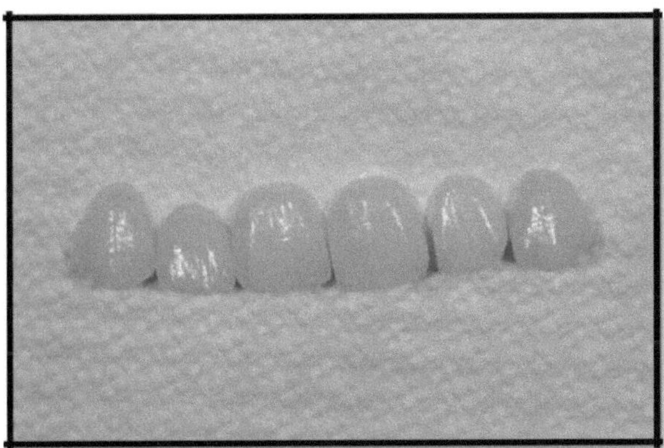

Figure 25

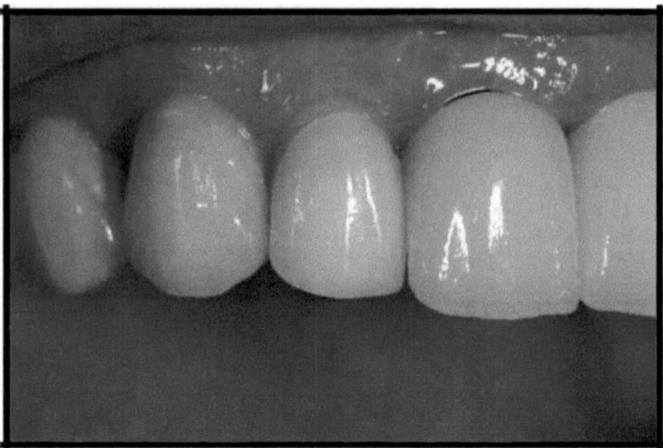

Figure 26

To prepare the veneers for definitive cementation, they were supported with addition silicon and then treated with 10% hydrofluoric acid for 60 seconds (Figure 27), washed thoroughly and dried (Figure 28), followed by application of Monobond Plus silane (Ivoclar-Vivadent) for 5 minutes (Figure 29). Finally, the adhesive system was applied to all the veneers without light curing (Figure 30).

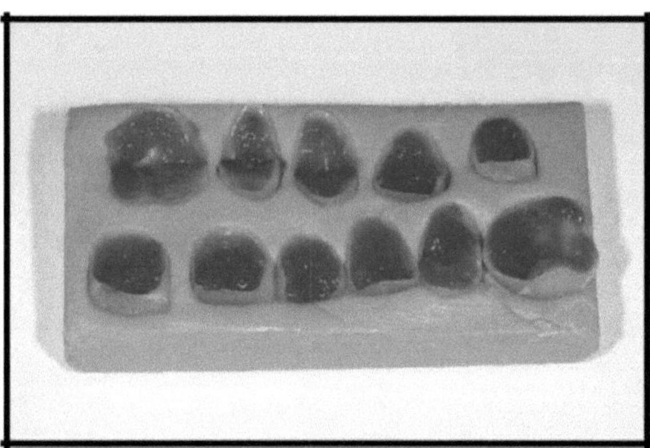

Figure 27

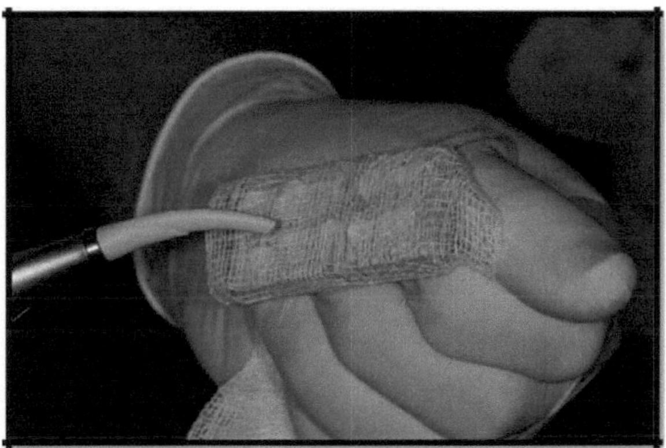

Figure 28

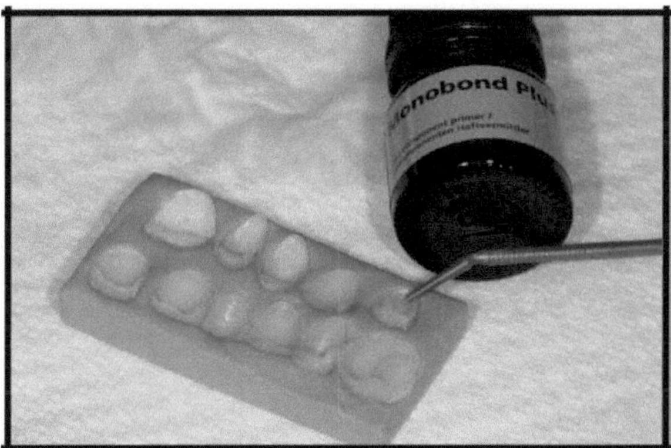

Figure 29

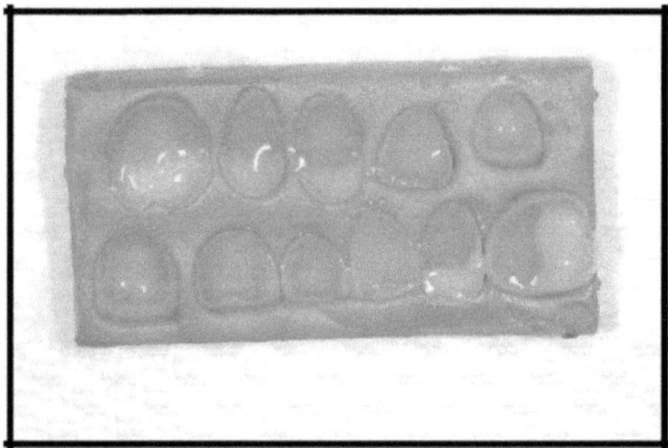

Figure 30

Treatment of the tooth preparations, using relative isolation, was carried out on the enamel with 37% phosphoric acid for 30 seconds (Figure 31), with abundant washing and drying (Figure 32) and application of the adhesive system, also without light curing (Figure 33).

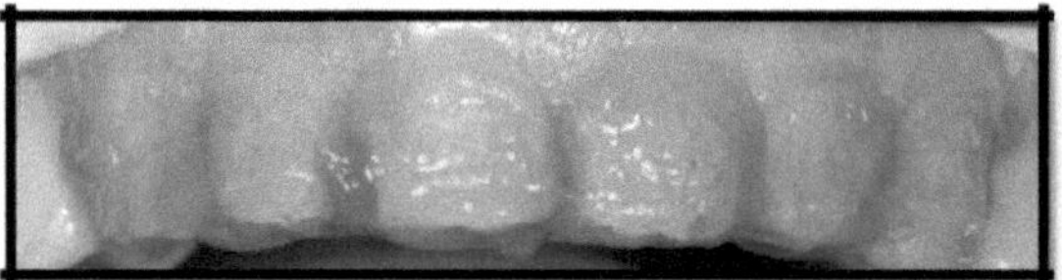

Figure 31

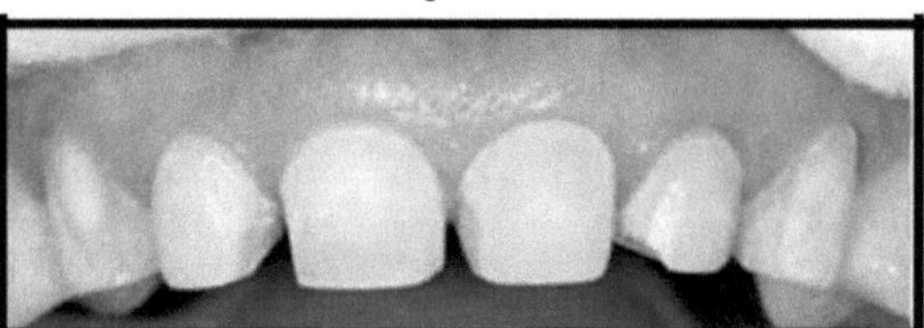

Figure 32

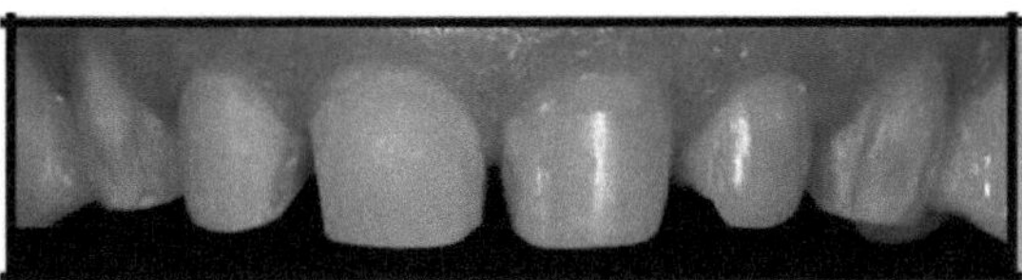

Figure 33

To complete the treatment, the veneers were permanently cemented with Variolink Venner light-curing cement in shade 110/A1 (White) and light-cured for one minute each (Figure 34; Figure 35).

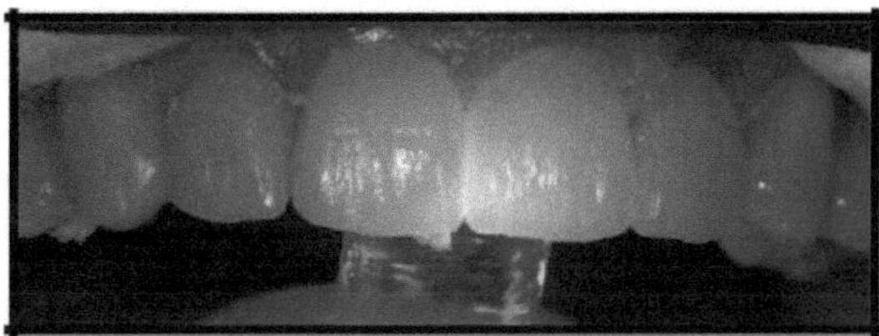

Figure 34

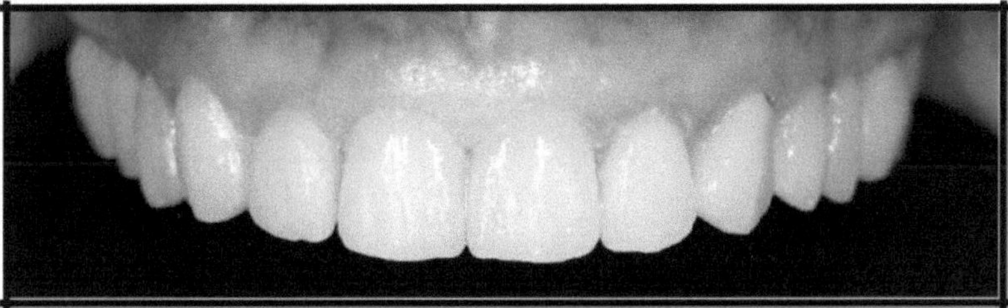

Figure 35

## 3. DISCUSSION

The first stage of the process is scanning the model, whose measurement method used by CEREC Omnicam (Sirona Dental Systems, Zurich, Germany) is active triangulation, which means measuring angles and depths, i.e. the camera projects a linear pattern under a triangulation angle of the cavity preparation and the image

is registered. When the preparation lines are visualised, the course of the lines no longer appears. At this stage, the lines do not appear flat, but are displaced locally, depending on the depth of tillage. The camera sensor registers these displacements and the software calculates the corresponding depth of preparation, allowing depths of 20 pm2 to be recorded. The 3D image generated is then transferred to CAD, where the system's SW 4.2 software allows the structures to be designed. The finishing line (definition of the margins) is detected automatically and can also be modified manually, which is then carried out on the system's milling machine (CAM)9.

Scanning with the CEREC Omnicam scanner can be carried out intra-orally or extra-orally. Intra-oral scanning allows for fewer clinical steps and also eliminates the possibility of distortion of the materials used in the moulding[4,10] . However, the extra-oral method is preferable[11] , as it allows for better reliability of the preparation, even with the disadvantages of time spent because it requires an impression of the dental preparation, which also introduces error factors into this process.

The software has a database where the anatomy of the teeth and prosthetic components are stored. When virtual waxing is required, the software assists the dental surgeon by inserting the image determined by the surgeon (veneers, crowns, etc.). As the CEREC system (Sirona Dental Systems, Zurich, Germany) is a closed system, it does not allow data to be sent or received by any other milling machines or systems .[10]

This system is capable of milling metal-free ceramic materials, particularly lithium disilicate1°, zirconia[3,12,13] and alumina[3] . Lithium disilicate metal free ceramic was chosen because of its aesthetics, translucency and high flexural strength.

The lithium disilicate crystals, created by adding lithium oxide to aluminium silicate glass, are densely arranged and bonded to a vitreous matrix in a proportion that varies from 60 to 70% by volume of crystals to glass matrix and are needle-shaped, which also contributes to the high flexural strength of this material, The CEREC MCXL milling unit (Sirona Dental Systems, Zurich, Germany) has four diamond drills that cut the block in four working axes with a reproducibility of approximately 30 pm5. The heat generated is controlled by constant water jets until the end of the separation process between the piece and the ceramic block, which is carried out by manual milling.

The disadvantage of the system is the possible cracks that can be generated by the milling process, which can jeopardise the mechanical performance of the prostheses. They occur more frequently when cooling is inadequate or when diamond tips are used several times and lose their cutting capacity .[17]

The use of the Try-In paste of Variolink Venner resin cement (Ivoclar-Vivadent, Germany) allows both the dental surgeon and the patient to assess the shade of the ceramic veneer, predicting the final aesthetics and providing predictability of the result .[18]

In this study, due to the use of an acid-sensitive ceramic, 10% hydrofluoric acid etching was carried out on the inner surface of the veneers. Its use is of great importance to increase the surface roughness of these ceramics, thus improving mechanical retention. However, the etching time and acid concentration are factors that must be controlled, respecting the time of 20 to 60 seconds[19,20,21,22,23] for lithium disilicate, otherwise partial dissolution may occur within the glassy matrix of the ceramic .[20]

Silane is the agent that ensures the chemical adhesion of the inorganic components of the ceramic to the organic portion of the resin cement. The purpose of applying silane to the ceramic surface, whether previously treated or not, is to improve the bond between the ceramic and the resin cement. It acts both physically, by increasing the wetting of the ceramic surface, making it more receptive to the adhesive, and chemically, by bonding it to the cement, similar to the bond between the inorganic particle and the organic matrix when composite resins are manufactured .[24]

Regarding the choice of cement for the definitive cementation of ceramic veneers, adhesive systems and photoactivated resin cements specifically designed for this purpose enable effective interaction between the ceramic and the dental structure

The use of exclusively photoactivated resin cements[27] is essential for maintaining aesthetics, colour stability of the ceramic veneer and better control of the positioning of the piece in the mouth, since they have the advantage of a longer working time, which makes it easier to remove excesses and less time for finishing[28] . The use of chemically activated cements is contraindicated[26,29] , as they may result in staining or colour alteration because they contain tertiary amine or benzoyl peroxide as a chemical activator, which can cause colour alterations over time and compromise the final aesthetic result .[30]

## 4. CONCLUSION

In the current phase of dentistry, CAD-CAM technology brings a new era of aesthetic restorative treatments, with better utilisation of professional time, reduced errors and increased quality through the use of automated techniques.

## 5. BIBLIOGRAPHICAL REFERENCES

1)  Witkowski S. (CAD-)/CAM in dental technology. Quintessence Dent Technol. 2005;28:169-84.

2)  Mormann WH. The origin of the Cerec method: a personal review of the first 5 years. Int J Comput Dent. 2004;7(1):11-24.

3)  Liu PR. A panorama of dental CAD/CAM restorative systems. Compendium. 2005;26:507-16.

4)  Duret F, Blouin JL, Duret B. CAD-CAM in dentistry. J Am Dent Assoc. 1988;(117):715-20.

5)  Sirona Denta Systems. Available at: http://www.sirona.com.br/br/produtos/ systems-cad-cam/cerec-chairside-solutions/. Accessed on 15 May 2015 at 14:45.

6)  Miyazaki T, Hotta Y, Kunii J, Kuriyama S, Tamaki Y. A review of dental CAD/CAM: current status and future perspectives from 20 years of experience. Dental Materials Journal. 2009;28(1):44-56.

7)  Mantri SS, Bhasin AS. CAD/CAM in dental restorations: an overview. Annals and Essences of Dentistry. 2010 July - Sept;2(3):123-28.

8)  Carvalho RLA, Faria JCB, Carvalho RF, Cruz FLG, Goyatá FR. Indications, marginal adaptation and clinical longevity of metal-free ceramic systems: a literature review. Int J Dent. 2012 January-Mar;11(1):55-65.

9)  Correia ARM, Sampaio Fernandes JCA, Cardoso JAP, Leal da Silva CFC. CAD-CAM: Information technology at the service of fixed prosthodontics. Revista de Odontologia da UNESP. 2006;35(2):183-89.

10)  Bernardes SR, Tiossi R, Mattias IAAM, Sartori GT. CAD/CAM technology applied to dental prostheses and implants: what it is, how it works, advantages and limitations. Critical review of the literature. ILAPEO Journal. 2012 January-February-March;6(1)

11) Tinschert J, Natt G, Hassenpflug S, Spiekermann H. Status of current CAD/CAM technology in dental medicine. International journal of computerised dentistry. 2004;7(1):25-45.

12) McLaren EA, Giordano RA. Zirconia-based ceramics: material properties, esthetics, and layering techniques of a new veneering porcelain. Quintessence Dent Technol. 2005;28:99-111.

13) Raigrodski AJ. Contemporary materials and technologies for all ceramic fixed partial dentures: a review of literature. The Journal of Prosthetic Dentistry. 2004;92(6):557-62.

14) Culp L, McLaren EA. Lithium disilicate: the restorative material of multiple options. Compendium. 2010 November-Dec;31(9):716-25.

15) Ritter RG, Rego NA. Material considerations for using lithium disilicate as a thin veneer option. Journal of Cosmetic Dentistry. 2009;25(3):111-7.

16) Priest G. Predictable Durability. Increasing All-Ceramic Treatment Durability in the Esthetic Zone Using Lithium Disillicate Restorations. Journal of Cosmetic Dentistry. 2011;27(2).

17) Fernandes CP. World Class Dentistry. Salvador, Santos Editora, 2010.

18) Cardoso PC, Lopes LG, de Souza JB. Importance of try-in paste in cementing ceramic veneers - Case Report. Robrac. 2011 Jul;20(53):166-71.

19) Borges GA, Sophr AM, De Goes MF, Sobrinho LC, Chan DC. Effect of etching and airborne particle abrasion on the microstructure of different dental ceramics, J Prosthet Dent. 2003 May;89(5):479-88.

20) Luo XP, Silikas N, Allaf M, Wilson NHF, Watts DC. AFM and SEM study of the effects of etching on IPS Empress 2tm dental ceramic, Surf Sci. 2001;491(3):388-94.

21) Meyer Filho A, Souza CN. Demystifying the adhesive cementation of ceramic restorations, Clínica: Internacional Journal Brazilian Dentistry. 2005;1(1):50-7.

22)  Nagai T, Kawamoto Y, Kakehashi Y, Matsumura H. Adhesive bonding of a lithium disilicate ceramic material with resin-based luting agents, Journal of Oral Rehabilitation. 2005 Aug;32(8):598-605.

23)  Camargo FP. Effect of thermal cycling on adhesion between a lithium disilicate ceramic and a resin cement. Pesquisa Odontológica Brasileira. 2002;16:83.

24)  Roulet JF, Soderholm KJM, Longmate J. Effects of treatment and storage conditions on ceramic/composite bond strength, Journal Dentistry Restorations. 1995 Jan;74(1):381-7.

25)  Lacy AM, LaLuz J, Watanabe LG, Dellinges M. Effect of porcelain surface treatment on the bond to composite. Journal Prosthetic Dentistry. 1988;60(3):288-91.

26)  Sensi L, Baratieri LN, Monteiro S Jr. Resin cements. In: Kina S, Bruguera A. Invisible: Aesthetic ceramic restorations. 1ª ed. Maringá: Dental Press; 2007:303-19.

27)  Guzman AF, Moore BK, Andres CJ. Wear resistance of four luting agents as a function of marginal gap distance, cement type, and restorative material. International Journal Prosthodontics. 1997 September-Oct;15(1):415-25.

28)  Peumans M, Van Meerbeek B, Yoshida Y, Lambrechts P, Vanherle G. Porcelain veneers bonded to tooth structure: an ultra morphological FE-SEM examination of the adhesive interface. Dent Mater. 1999 Mar;15(2):105-19.

29)  Karaaglioglu, L., Yilmaz, B. Influence of cement shade and water storage on the final colour of leucite-reinforced ceramics.*Oper. Dent.* 2008;33(4):386-91

30)  Aquino APT, Cardoso PC, Rodrigues MB, Takano AE, Porfirio W. Porcelain Veneers: Aesthetic and Functional Solution. International Journal of Brazilian Dentistry. 2009;5(2):142-52.

ELOISA ANDRADE DE PAULA

DANIELLI ANTONIO SCHUARZ

# DIFFERENCES IN RESTORATIVE PLANNING BETWEEN CONTACT LENSES AND VENEERS: LITERATURE REVIEW.

CASCAVEL
2015

# SUMMARY

In recent years, the dental surgeon has been faced with a high degree of aesthetic demand from patients who are increasingly looking for aligned, whitened teeth that fit into a harmonious pattern. Aesthetics is the dominant factor in planning anterior prosthetic rehabilitation, without neglecting function. Currently, with the development of aesthetic restorative materials associated with adhesive techniques, it is possible to make extremely thin restorations 0.3 to 0.5 mm thick, called ultra thin ceramic laminates (UFTCL), with high resistance, supported by adhesive cementation. However, these materials are not always able to mask the colour of the underlying tooth structure, making it necessary to use conventional ceramic laminates or veneers with a thickness of 0.5 mm in the cervical area, 0.7 mm in the middle and incisal thirds and more than 1.5 mm of coverage. The aim of this study was to review the literature on the indications and contraindications of veneers and LCUF and to discuss the different aspects related to rehabilitative treatment with ceramics.

**Key words:** ceramics, aesthetics, dental veneers.

**INTRODUCTION**

The incessant search for beauty standards makes people look for treatments that offer the perfect smile. Aesthetic dentistry is continually advancing due to adhesive procedures and the development of restorative materials that seek to reproduce the natural characteristics of dental structures (SILVA et al., 2014).

Until the mid-1980s, prosthetic treatment options were called metal-ceramic, where the crown is formed by a metal base "coping" covered with ceramic. First came feldspathic porcelain, which had low tensile and fracture strengths. These properties were compensated for with the emergence of resin cements used during cementation, providing adhesion of the piece to the dental structure (CARDOSO et al., 2011).

With evolution, reinforced ceramics have been created, with the addition of crystals such as alumina, leucite, lithium disilicate and zirconia increasing resistance, making it possible to replace metal coping (not aesthetic) and making minimally invasive, thin laminates with high longevity and better aesthetic results (CARDOSO et al., 2011).

The first report in the literature of the use of ceramic laminates or veneers appeared in 1928 when Holywood actors used them for filming (BISPO, 2009). The use of veneers became popular in 1983, with the work of Horn and Simonsen and Calamia, who developed the technique of acid etching porcelain, which made it possible to make restorations fixed to tooth preparations with no form of retention and therefore dependent on a strong ceramic/resin/tooth bond (CALAMIA et al., 1984).

As the technique evolved, porcelain veneers began to be referred to as ultra-thin ceramic laminates (UCTL) and, as this is a relatively new term, there are various definitions in the literature such as contact lenses due to their similarity in thinness to ophthalmological contact lenses (BARATIERI et al., 2015), ultra-conservative ceramic laminates, minimally invasive ceramic fragments and thin venners.), ultraconservative, minimally invasive ceramic laminates, ceramic fragments and "thin venners", which are indicated for closing interdental diastemas, small changes in shape and position, adding volume to the dental element, incisal length and added to teeth in order to modify or restore their original shape (MELLO CC. et al.,2012) (MAZARO et al., 2009).

The main indications for veneers are the same as for LCUF, but changes to the shape, position and alignment of the tooth in the arch should require greater wear of the tooth structure, as well as colour correction where whitening treatment has not been satisfactory and smile rehabilitation cases.

However, with the popularisation of the technique, there is a need to define the correct indication and preparation protocols to guide professionals in clinical practice as to the limitations of each treatment. The aim of this study is to describe the differences in the indication of the two aesthetic restorative treatments: veneers and LCUF, as well as the variations in preparation methods, difficulties and limitations of the techniques and the differences in adhesive cementation.

## LITERATURE REVIEW

### Evolution of ceramic laminates

Ceramics were used as a dental material for the first time in 1774 to make teeth for full dentures by chemist Alexis Duchateau and dentist Nicholas Dubois. Later, new ways of handling ceramics were patented and the manufacture of all-ceramic crowns on a platinum veneer was realised with the invention of the electric furnace (1894) and low-fusion porcelain (1898) (BADER etal.,2009).

In 1886, Charles Henry Land made the first ceramic restoration on a prepared tooth (Metzler, K., 1999) using a sheet of platinum (MONDELLI and CONEGLIAN, 2003). Porcelain as an aesthetic resource began in the 20th century when film stars needed to improve the harmony of their smiles. Dr Charles Pincus created the technique of covering aesthetically compromised teeth with a porcelain veneer provisionally bonded with powder for fixing full dentures and lasting as long as necessary for the recording, since he had not mastered the cementation technique (SOUZA et al., 2002).

From the 1950s onwards, leucite was added to the formulation of dental ceramics, thus increasing their resistance without interfering with the opacity of the piece (RADZ et al.,2011). In the 1960s Mc Lean introduced feldspathic porcelain reinforced with aluminium oxide particles, but ceramic laminates only became popular in the 1980s (SPEAR,2008).

In 1975, Alain Rochette was the first to describe the use of adhesive ceramic restorations in anterior teeth. This author published the technique for rehabilitating fractured incisors using unconditioned silanised ceramic cemented to acid-conditioned enamel using acrylic resin.

It wasn't until 1983 that ceramic veneers came to the fore as a restorative option, when Simonsen and Calamina described the conditioning of ceramics with 10% hydrofluoric acid, similar to the acid used to condition dental enamel (SIMONSEN ET.AL 1983).

In the same year, it was reported that the ceramic veneer was the treatment indicated to mask fractures, irregularities and diastemas (HORN, H., 1983). Its advantages over the existing direct composite veneer treatment were: less staining, resistance to the deleterious effects of alcohol, medications and solvents and greater adhesion effectiveness.

With the evolution of materials and techniques in dentistry, as well as the advent of adhesive retention, extremely conservative tooth preparations have been adopted, with minimal wear or, depending on the case, even no preparation at all. The development of reinforced ceramic pieces has made it possible to make very thin veneers, with a thickness of between 0.3 and 0.5 mm, which are known as LCUF.

Currently, veneer restorations are considered predictable in terms of longevity, periodontal response and patient satisfaction (SHETTY et al., 2011), as well as being the main alternative restorative material for the dental structure due to their properties such as: resistance to compression, thermal conductivity, similarity to dental tissues, radiopacity, marginal integrity, colour stability, biomimicry, among others. The demand for aesthetic restorations has resulted in an increase in the use of dental ceramics, which used to be restricted to treatment in anterior regions, but now also covers the posterior region (RAUT, 2011).

## Veneers

Veneers are partial restorations designed to cover the buccal, proximal and incisal surfaces of anterior teeth (BISPO, 2009). They are divided into direct veneers, which are made by the professional himself using composite resins or prefabricated veneers, and indirect veneers, which are made by the prosthodontist using indirect resins or porcelain (SOUZA et al., 2002). The recommended thicknesses for porcelain veneers are less than 0.5 mm in the cervical area, 0.7 mm in the middle and incisal thirds and more than 1.5 mm of incisal coverage (MAGNE, 2007).

The indication for veneers arose at a time when there was a great deal of questioning about the use of invasive techniques, such as subjecting patients to tooth wear to make full crowns, or other aesthetic procedures that involved a great deal of tissue loss (BERGENHOLZT, 1984).

Veneers can be indicated when problems arise (SILVA e SOUZA et al. 1995; HAGA & NAKAZAWA, 1995; MAGNE and BELSER, 2003):

- Shape;
- Position and alignment;
- Symmetry and proportion;
- Surface texture and colour;
- Microdontics;
- Teeth that do not respond to internal and external whitening;
- Conical teeth and malformed teeth - naturally present an ideal configuration for the use of veneers, requiring only a slight marginal chamfer to give strength to the ceramic piece;
- Diastemas and gyroversions;
- Teeth discoloured by devitalisation*;
- Teeth altered in colour by restorations;
- Teeth that have changed colour due to medication (tetracycline, fluoride)*;
- Teeth with abrasion or attrition*; 'indications with limitations.

## Indications with limitations

Tetracycline discolouration should always be done at home first and, if the result is unsatisfactory, then veneers should be used. It is common for veneers to fail to mask stains and give an unnatural appearance, but due to the increasingly better performance of dentin adhesives, deeper preparations can be carried out to improve the final result.

With the emergence of new materials and techniques, it became possible to indicate veneers in compromising situations, making it possible to cover the incisal edge (including extensive class IV preparations up to fractures in the middle third) and proximal enveloping.

Veneers are also suitable for endodontically treated teeth, as they can substantially increase coronal mechanical strength and restore the original rigidity of the tooth, especially when the ceramic is thick enough to reproduce the original volume and length of the crown.

Isolated cases of diastema closure can be treated with direct composite resins, but multiple diastemas are best resolved with porcelain veneers, which make it easier to achieve colour, contour, emergence profile and cervical adaptation.

Extensive dental abrasion is typically found in older people, but young people are increasingly affected by this problem due to the greater presence of acids in the diet. Conservative treatments are used, such as rinsing with sodium bicarbonate solutions and topical application of neutral fluoride gels, before considering the use of composite resins or veneers, which will depend on the extent of the wear.

All indications prioritise aesthetics and restoring the form and function of the tooth, provided that the other portions of the tooth, such as the palatal region, are healthy or poorly restored.

**Limitations**

Consider the limitations that are important for the safe prognosis of ceramic veneers (BARATIERI et al., 2001):
- Failure to preserve at least 50% of the buccal enamel and also when the margins are not enamelled;
- Endodontically treated teeth with colour change;
- Patients with parafunctional habits and inadequate occlusion;
- Teeth with short or excessively thin clinical crowns in the incisal region;
- Patients with high caries activity;
- Teeth with multiple or wide restorations.

**Preparation**

In order to carry out an adequate preparation that provides the conditions for a resistant, stable and aesthetically excellent piece, it is necessary to follow a previous protocol. Below we will describe what is suggested by (BARATIERI et al.,2001):

- Making silicone guides - to prevent excessive enamel wear and promote uniform wear (Magne and Belser). The guide is made directly in the patient's mouth when the enamel thickness of the teeth is unchanged, or on a study model when a diagnostic wax-up is indicated.

- Use a chemical-free retractor wire compatible with the depth of the gingival sulcus. Shallow grooves and thin gingival margins use #00 and #000 floss, deep grooves and thicker gingival margins use #0 and #1 floss, especially in cases of subgingival preparations, to facilitate visibility, taking care not to overextend the preparation, as the reference may be lost due to the floss.

- The preparation should begin by making a groove in the cervical region with a 1011 or 1012 diamond tip. The depth of the groove will vary according to the degree of darkening of the tooth and the need to replace the enamel according to the silicone guide of around 0.5 mm. The chamfered preparation is proving to be the best form of cervical termination for successful work with laminates, enabling correct marginal adaptation, resin cement flow and being very favourable for delimiting the limits of the preparation.

- Creation of a central groove following the inclination of the crown, using a 4138 conical truncated diamond point with a rounded end, at high speed. The depth of this groove depends on the same factors mentioned above, as well as the degree of inclination, but the depth varies around 0.7 mm.

- With the same tapered stem tip, the distal half and then the mesial half of the buccal surface should be worn down.

- For the proximal preparation, it is important to protect the adjacent teeth with a metal strip and, above all, to consider the contact areas, so as not to allow tooth structure with altered colouring in this location to become visible after the veneer has been cemented. If the tooth has proximal restorations with caries lesions, these should be involved in the preparation (they should be removed). Whenever possible, the proximal contacts should be kept in natural tooth, as this region has anatomical characteristics that are difficult to reproduce; they reduce the risk of tooth movement; they make it easier to adjust the veneers; they simplify adhesion and finishing procedures; they facilitate plaque control.

- Four types of preparation of the incisal region are carried out: the "window" preparation, limited to the buccal side of the tooth; the "enveloped" preparation, with wear of the palatal side of the incisal third with a small 0.5mm chamfer (the most traditional preparation but one that is being carried out less these days); wear of the palatal side of the incisal third without a chamfer finish; and wear of the incisal third without preservation of the structure, of approximately 1.0 mm.

- The literature cites four other types of preparation that are used for incisal reduction, which are defined as 0°, straight, 45° and chamfer. The clinical recommendations are: 0° ceramic fragments and ceramic restorations without preparation; straight and 45° conventional ceramic restorations or without preparation; and chamfer conventional ceramic restorations specific to: very thin incisal thickness, the need to reconstitute 1.0 to 2.0 mm of restorative material volume in the incisal, the presence of structurally compromised incisal enamel and individuals with parafunction (BARATIERI et al., 2015).

- Subgingival preparation is indicated in cases of endodontic treatment with colour change, this extension is required to mask the termination by about 0.2 mm. When there is no need for subgingival preparation, the termination can be kept supra-gingivally, or at the level of the gingival margin, with the following advantages:

-easy to determine the form of the termination;

-easy to visualise the finish line;

-simplification of moulding procedures;

-favouring the fit check in this critical area:

-decreased risk of contamination during adhesive cementing procedures;
-Easy to visualise and remove excess resin cement;

-simplification of the finishing and polishing steps;

-easy to clean;

-ease of monitoring "margin behaviour" over time.

After completing the preparation with the diamond tips, it is important to use a sequence of flexible abrasive discs, such as Sof-Lex, to refine and help round off the angles of the preparation, aiding the properties and seating of the veneer after cementation (MAGNE and BELSER, 2003).

Among the various preparation techniques, the objective is always the same, comprising: maximum preservation of healthy tooth structures, the principles of retention and stability, the characteristics of solidity or structural strength of the restorative materials, marginal integrity and preservation of the periodontium.

**Ultra-thin ceramic laminates**

They are very thin ceramic sheets (0.3 to 0.5 mm) that cover the entire face of the tooth (vestibular) and can be made without any wear, or when necessary, only retentive areas that could jeopardise the insertion of the ceramic pieces are removed. LCUFs are durable due to their adhesion to enamel and less bending of the tooth structure due to the preservation of structures that provide mechanical resistance to the tooth (BARATIERI et al., 2015).

Indicated in situations where the tooth position allows for the addition of material, because even if tooth wear is necessary, it should be minimal, limited to enamel (it is essential that as much enamel as possible is preserved). Examples of indications are listed below (BARATIERI et al., 2015):

- Incisal edge augmentation - When there is a fracture or wear and reconstruction of the original shape is required. This indication also applies to the incisal edge of canines, with the aim of restoring lateral occlusal protection guides, provided that the patient has undergone orthodontic rehabilitation treatment.

- Closing diastemas - Whenever it is necessary to re-contour the teeth, respecting the natural proportion. These situations are often encountered in patients who have had orthodontic treatment.

- Volume gain and conoid teeth - In cases where we need to expand the patient's arch so that the smile is more harmonious with the labial commissure or so that we have a smile with a perspective of continuity between the front and back teeth. This indication also applies to teeth that are in a palatal or lingual position and need to be buccalised.

**Limitations**

- Need for extensive wear of the tooth structure.
- Teeth with a pronounced buccal profile.
- Blackened teeth.
- Unfavourable insertion axis.

**Preparation**

Whenever possible, wear and tear on tooth structure should be avoided in order to carry out LCUF, as the greater the amount of tooth tissue removed, the lower the strength of the tooth.

The decision whether or not to wear down the tooth structure is guided by three aspects that must be assessed with the help of initial photographs and the diagnostic wax-up:
- Possibility of adding material;
- Axis for inserting parts;
- Whether or not to mask the colour of the dental substrate;

Although Baratieri et al. 2015 suggest that preparations for LCUF depend on each case, i.e. there is no specific preparation, only the removal of convexities, angles or minimal terminations, Pascal Magne and Michel Magne suggest that preparations be made in the cervical and interproximal regions of the tooth, that terminations be made with a small chamfer and without very demarcated angles on the internal line, in order to improve the adhesion of the ceramic-tooth complex (PASCAL MAGNE AND MICHEL MAGNE, 2005).

When planning indicates the need for tooth wear, this can occur in the following ways:
- **Visual:** The retentive areas of the tooth structure that must be removed in order to establish the insertion axis of the ceramic restorations are demarcated with a pencil or pen.
- **Guided by the silicone guide:** Removal of the retainers and measurement of the spaces obtained are carried out using silicone guides based on the diagnostic wax-up.

**Moulding**

Moulding is usually carried out immediately after the preparation procedures have been completed, so it is important to avoid the slightest trauma to the gingival tissue.

The material of choice is addition silicon because it has excellent dimensional stability and can be stored for up to 14 days before pouring, it has reproduction fidelity and elastic recovery, and it also allows double pouring of the model, the first for the die mould and the second for adjusting the proximal contacts. It should be noted that this model should not be poured before 2 hours, as the release of chemical reaction products from this material could affect the quality of the model. The second option for moulding material is polyethers (SOUZA et al., 2002; HIRATA et al., 1999; VELEDA et al., 2011).

For veneers, Magne and Belser (2003) propose the use of a small diameter wire, which will remain in the groove during moulding, sealing the groove and limiting the fluid. A second, larger diameter wire is then inserted and removed during the moulding process. This retraction should be carried out for at least five to ten minutes before the impression is taken, in order to allow the retractor wire to expand through water absorption (MAGNE AND BELSER, 2003). Retractor wires should be used to keep the copy of the cervical part true, avoiding gaps (SOUZA et al., 2002). The surface must be dry, especially if the preparation is subgingival. The moulding can be made with the small diameter wire in position or by removing it (HIRATA et al.,1999).

After removing the wire, the light moulding material is placed inside the groove, pressed into the groove with a light jet of air, and the tray is inserted, preferably a full tray loaded with a more viscous material. The professional handling the heavy material should not wear gloves and should have clean hands to avoid contaminating the material.

The tray is removed from the mouth, rinsed and analysed thoroughly to assess the quality of the impression. The moulding must be perfect so that there are no problems when trying on the veneer (MAGNE E BALSER et al., 2003).

The success of the moulding is directly linked to a well-made preparation, which must be smooth and polished (VELEDA et al., 2011).

All of the above refers to moulding for both veneers and LCUF, but the biggest difference between them is that in LCUF, the retractor wire should not be used, as the gingival distance alters the reference of the gingival tissues in relation to the delicate end of the cervical preparation, which can result in pieces with a cervical overcontour (BARATIERI etal.,2015).

**Materials**

It advocates the use of conditionable ceramic systems due to their high aesthetic properties (BARATIERI et al., 2015).

- **Vitablocs® (vita):**
  - Feldspathic ceramics. CAD/CAM processing.
  - Excellent aesthetics.
  - They are fragile.
  - Compressive strength is high, while tensile strength is low.
  - A huge variety of colours, shades, values, pigments and translucency characteristics, making it possible to reproduce many of the chromatic details of neighbouring natural teeth.
  - Suitable for veneers and LCUF on anterior teeth, cover ceramics on single or multiple dentures and partial restorations on posterior teeth.

- **IPS Empress® ceramic system (ivoclar vivadent):**
There are two forms of processing: leucite-reinforced glass-ceramic, processed by injection under heat and pressure, and CAD/CAM.
- resistance index is higher than feldspathic, favouring the indication of multiple rehabilitation.
- They are suitable for veneers and LCUF on anterior teeth, cover ceramics on single or multiple prostheses and partial restorations on posterior teeth.

- **e.max® Press/ e.max® CAD (Ivoclar vivadent)**
There are two ways of processing lithium disilicate reinforced glass ceramics by injection moulding under heat and pressure.
- Superior resistance.
- Excellent aesthetics.
- They are suitable for ultra-thin ceramic laminates to 3-element fixed prostheses.
- They are substitutes for the indications for leucite-reinforced ceramics.

**Colour selection**

Colour registration can be selected using the vita scale and also by means of photographs that are sent to the ceramist to observe the details of colour and shape of the dental elements to be reproduced (HIRATA et al., 2004).

Chiche and Pinault (1996) indicated that natural light should be preferred for colour selection, stains and deposits should be removed from the tooth surface and the tooth should be kept moist. They point out that the first impression is very important, as spontaneity usually gives the best results, but if you are not sure which colour to select, you should not look at the tooth for more than 20 seconds, as you will lose sensitivity to yellow. In this case, it is advisable to look at green or blue objects to rest the eye (CHICHE and PINAULT,1996).

Colour selection should be avoided after anaesthesia, after preparation or after a very painful appointment. It is interesting to note the variations in colour of the same tooth between the cervical, middle and incisal thirds, as well as the appearance of the nipples and incisal translucency (CHICHE, 1996).

**Cementing**

- Proofing **the pieces** - Prior to the cementation stage, the tooth structure should be prophylaxed and the ceramic pieces proofed. Prophylaxis should be carried out with a pumice stone and a rubber cup or Robson brush. Care should be taken in the proximal areas, as this is where biofilm accumulates most. When testing, the insertion axis and contact point should be observed.

- **Surface treatment -** Start the treatment by applying 10% hydrofluoric acid to the inside of the part. After the conditioning time, the acid is removed under running water. After washing and drying, you will find a white, opaque surface, which are debris from the etching. These should be removed by immersion in an ultrasonic tank for 5 minutes, or by active application of 37% phosphoric acid using a microbrush, followed by rinsing again with running water.

  The silane is applied to the conditioned surface. This is followed by drying, application of the adhesive system in a thin layer and drying again. On the tooth structure, after prophylaxis with a pumice stone, etching should be carried out with 37% phosphoric acid for 30s on the enamel, followed by rinsing with a water jet and air drying. The adhesive system will be applied to the duly conditioned tooth surface, an air jet will be applied to evaporate the solvent and light-curing will take place (BARATIERI et al., 2015).

- **Cementation itself -** An exclusively light-curing resin cement must be applied to the piece and the tooth structure. The piece is then seated on the tooth, one at a time, and excess cement is removed using brushes, dental floss and an exploratory probe. Light-curing is then carried out (BARATIERI et al., 2015).

## CONCLUSION

A correct knowledge of veneer and LCUF techniques is essential for treatment planning and execution. The main indications for veneers are the same as for LCUFs, but changes to the shape, position and alignment of the tooth require greater wear of the tooth structure.

The LCUF preparation should be conservative and preserve the tooth structure as much as possible, while in veneer cases it is indicated in cases of greater need for wear. The material of choice for the moulding procedure is addition silicone in both treatments. The only difference in this protocol is the use of the retractor wire, which in LCUF cases is not used so as not to alter the reference of the gingival tissues.

In view of the above, it can be concluded that the dental surgeon needs to have knowledge of both techniques, as correct indication is essential for carrying out the treatment.

# BIBLIOGRAPHICAL REFERENCES

1. BADER JD, SHUGARS, DA. Summary review of the survival of single crowns, **General Dentistry.** v.57, n.1, p.74-81,2009.

2. BARATIERI, L. N. et al. Restorative Dentistry - **Fundamentals and Possibilities.** 1.ed. São Paulo. Ed. Santos, 2001.

3. BARATIERI, N. L. et al. **Restorative Dentistry: Fundamentals and Possibilities.** 2.ed. São Paulo: Santos, 2015. p.852.

4. BENETTI, A. R. et al. Indirect Porcelain Veneers: Aesthetic Alternative. **Jornal Brasileiro de Dentistica e Estética**, Curitiba, v.2, n.7, p.186-194, jul./set. 2003.

5. BISPO, L. B. Aesthetic Veneers: Status of the Art. **Revista Dentistica on line,** v.8, n.18. jan./mar. 2009.

6. CALAMIA, J. R.; SIMONSEN, R. J. Effect of coupling agents on bond strength of etched porcelain. **Journal of Dental Research,** Washington, v.63, p.162- 362, Mar.1984.

7. CALICCHIO, L. et al. **Precision: the secrets of minimally invasive aesthetic dentistry.** São Paulo: Quintessence, 2014. p.173.

8. CARDOSO, P. C. et al. Functional aesthetic restoration with ceramic laminates. **Revista odontológica do brasil central (ROBRAC),** Goiânia, v.20, n.52, p.88-93, 2011.

9. CHICHE, J. P.; PINAULT, A. Aesthetics in anterior fixed prostheses. **Quintessence Editora,** 1996.

10. CULP, L.; MCLAREN, E. A. Lithium disilicate: the restorative material of multiple options. Compendium v.31, n.9, p.716-725, Nov./Dec. 2010

11. FERNANDES, M.G. et al. Indirect aesthetic restorations: clinical case reports. **Clínica-Cientifica,** Recife, v.6, n.4, p.329-333, Oct./Dec. 2007.

12. GROVER, V. R. C. et al. IPS e.Max: harmonising the smile. **Revista Dental Press de Estética**, Maringá , v.4, n.1, p.33-49, 2007.

13. HAGA, M; NAKAZAWA, A. Technique for making porcelain laminate veneers.l.ed. São Paulo: Santos, 1995.

14. HIRATA, R.; CARNIEL, C. Z. Solving some common clinical problems with the use of direct and indirect veneers: a broad vision. **Brazilian Journal of Clinical & Aesthetic Dentistry,** v.3, n.15, p.7-17, 2004.

15. HIRATA, R. et al. Clinical Alternatives for Composite Resin Systems

Laboratory Tests: When and How to Use Them. **Brazilian Journal of Clinical & Aesthetics in Dentistry,** v.4, n.19, p.13-21,2000.

16. KELLY,JR, BENETTI, P. Ceramic materials in dentistry: historical evolution and current practice. **Australian Dental Journal,** v.56 n.1, p.84-96, 2011.

17. KINA, S. Dental ceramics. **Dental Press Journal of Aesthetics,** v.2, n.2, p.112-28, 2005.

18. KINA,S. et al. Ceramic Laminates. **Aesthetic Dentistry - The State of the Art.** São Paulo: Artes Médicas, p.181-201, 2004.

19. MAGNE, P and MAGNE, M. Treatment of extended anterior crown fractures using type IIIA bonded porcelain restorations. **J Calif Dent Assoe,** v.33, n.5, p.387-396, 2005.

20. MAGNE, P. Use of Addition Closure and Intraoral Direct Trial for Enamel Preservation with Porcelain Laminate Veneers. **Revista Clinica: International journal of brazilian dentistry,** São José, v.3 n.1, p.25-31. Jan/Mar 2007.

21. MAGNE, P.; BELSER, U. Adhesive Porcelain Restorations in the Anterior Dentition - A Biomimetic Approach. São Paulo: Quintessence Ed., 2003.

22. MAZARRO, J. V. Q. et al. Clinical considerations for the restoration of the anterior region with laminate veneers. **Revista Odontológica de Araçatuba,** Araçatuba, v.30, n.1, p.48-51, jan./jun. 2009.

23. MELLO,CC. et al. Minimally invasive aesthetic treatment: contact lenses. **Araçatuba School of Dentistry,** May 2012.

24. MENDES, W.P. et al. Laminate Veneers - Ceramic and Resin: clinical aspects. **Book of the Year of the Brazilian Dental Clinic,** São Paulo: Artes Médicas, v.2, p. 27-59, 2004.

25. METZLER, K., et al. (1999). In Vitro Investigation of the Wear of Human Enamel by Dental Porcelain. **Journal of Prosthetic Dentistry,** v.81, n.3, p.356-64.

26. MONDELLI, R. F. L.; CONEGLIAN, E. A. C.; MONDELLI, J. Aesthetic rehabilitation of the smile with indirect porcelain veneers. **Revista Biodonto,** São Paulo, v.1, n.5, Sep/Oct 2003.

27. PINCUS, C. Building Mouth Personality. **Journal of the California Dental Association,** v.14, p.125-129, 1938.

28. RAUT A. et al. Zirconium for aesthetic rehabilitation: an overview. **Indian Journal of Dental,** v.22, n.1, p.140-3, 2011.

29. SHETTY, A. et al. Survival rates of porcelain laminate restoration based on different incisal preparation designs. **Journal of Conservative Dentistry.** v.14, p.10-

15,2011.

30. SILVA E SOUZA et.al(1995)-souza EM. de silva e Souza JR. Et al. Indirect aesthetic porcelain veneers. **Brazilian Journal of Clinical Dentistry.** Curitiba, v.1, n.3, p.256-262,jul./set/2012.

31. SOUZA, E. M. et al. Indirect aesthetic porcelain veneers. **Brazilian Journal of Clinical Dentistry,** Curitiba, v. 1, n. 3, p. 256-62, jul./set. 2002.

32. TEIXEIRA, H. M.; NASCIMENTO, A. B. L.; AMERICANO, M. Rehabilitation of aesthetics with indirect porcelain veneers. **Jornal Brasileiro Dentistica Estética,** Curitiba, v.2, n.7, p. 219-223, Sep/Oct 2003.

33. VELEDA, B. B; MELARA, R. Re-anatomisation of anterior teeth with ceramic laminates: clinical case report. 2011. Monograph (Specialisation) - Federal University of Rio Grande do Sul, Porto Alegre, 2011.

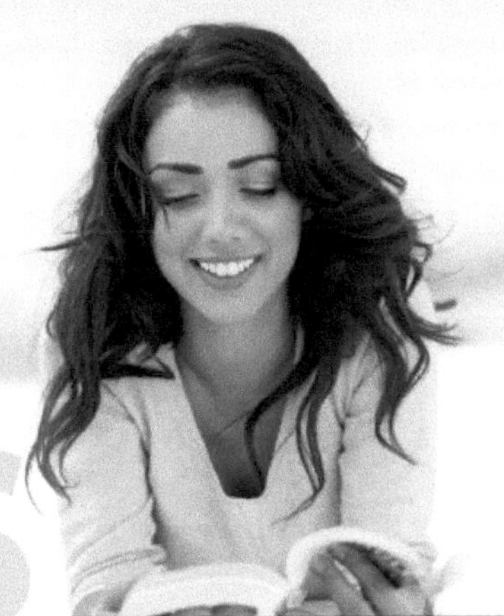

# I want morebooks!

Buy your books fast and straightforward online - at one of world's fastest growing online book stores! Environmentally sound due to Print-on-Demand technologies.

Buy your books online at
## www.morebooks.shop

Kaufen Sie Ihre Bücher schnell und unkompliziert online – auf einer der am schnellsten wachsenden Buchhandelsplattformen weltweit! Dank Print-On-Demand umwelt- und ressourcenschonend produziert.

Bücher schneller online kaufen
## www.morebooks.shop

info@omniscriptum.com
www.omniscriptum.com

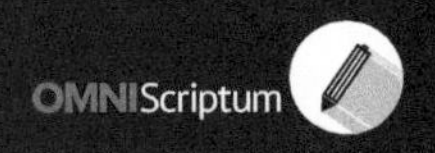

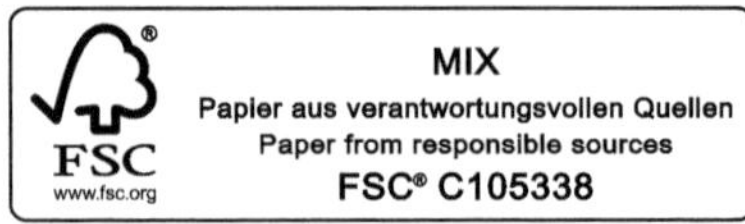

Printed by Books on Demand GmbH, Norderstedt / Germany